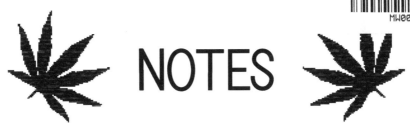 NOTES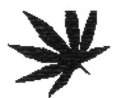

STRAIN

Grower _____ Date _____

Acquired _____ $ _____

THC Amount _____	CBD Oil Amount _____	☐ Indica	☐ Hybrid	☐ Sativa

☐ Flower   ☐ Edible   ☐ Concentrate

Symptoms Relieved

_____

_____

_____

_____

Consumed Method

Smoke	Ate	Vape	External
Rolled	Butter	Pen	Patch
Pipe	Gum		Cream
Water Pipe	Drink		Other
Blunt	Edibles		_____
Dabbed	Tincture		_____
	Oil		_____

Try Again ☐ Yes   ☐ No

Sweet
Fruity
Floral
Sour
Spicy
Earthy
Herbal
Woodsy

Effects	Strength				
Peaceful	○	○	○	○	○
Sleepy	○	○	○	○	○
Pain Relief	○	○	○	○	○
Hungry	○	○	○	○	○
Uplifted	○	○	○	○	○
Creative	○	○	○	○	○

Rating

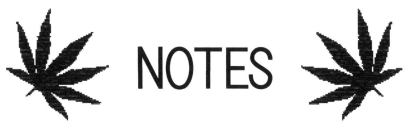

NOTES

STRAIN

Grower _____ Date _____

Acquired _____ $ _____

| THC Amount _____ | CBD Oil Amount _____ | ☐ Indica | ☐ Hybrid | ☐ Sativa |

☐ Flower   ☐ Edible   ☐ Concentrate

Symptoms Relieved

_____

_____

_____

_____

Consumed Method

Smoke	Ate	Vape	External
Rolled	Butter	Pen	Patch
Pipe	Gum		Cream
Water Pipe	Drink		Other
Blunt	Edibles		_____
Dabbed	Tincture		_____
	Oil		_____

Try Again ☐ Yes   ☐ No

Aroma Wheel
Sweet, Fruity, Floral, Sour, Spicy, Earthy, Woodsy, Herbal

Effects	Strength
Peaceful	○ ○ ○ ○ ○
Sleepy	○ ○ ○ ○ ○
Pain Relief	○ ○ ○ ○ ○
Hungry	○ ○ ○ ○ ○
Uplifted	○ ○ ○ ○ ○
Creative	○ ○ ○ ○ ○

Rating 🌿 🌿 🌿 🌿 🌿

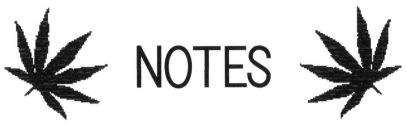

NOTES

STRAIN

Grower _____   Date _____

Acquired _____ $ _____

| THC Amount _____ | CBD Oil Amount _____ | ☐ Indica | ☐ Hybrid | ☐ Sativa |

☐ Flower   ☐ Edible   ☐ Concentrate

Symptoms Relieved

_____

_____

_____

_____

Consumed Method

Smoke	Ate	Vape	External
Rolled	Butter	Pen	Patch
Pipe	Gum		Cream
Water Pipe	Drink		Other
Blunt	Edibles		_____
Dabbed	Tincture		_____
	Oil		_____

Try Again   ☐ Yes   ☐ No

Sweet
Fruity   Floral
Sour   ●   Spicy
Earthy   Herbal
Woodsy

Effects	Strength				
Peaceful	○	○	○	○	○
Sleepy	○	○	○	○	○
Pain Relief	○	○	○	○	○
Hungry	○	○	○	○	○
Uplifted	○	○	○	○	○
Creative	○	○	○	○	○

Rating 🌿 🌿 🌿 🌿 🌿

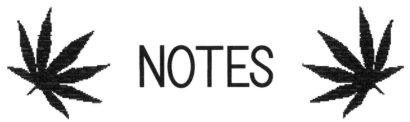

NOTES

STRAIN

Grower _____   Date _____

Acquired _____ $ _____

| THC Amount _____ | CBD Oil Amount _____ | ☐ Indica | ☐ Hybrid | ☐ Sativa |

☐ Flower   ☐ Edible   ☐ Concentrate

Symptoms Relieved

_____

_____

_____

_____

Consumed Method

Smoke	Ate	Vape	External
Rolled	Butter	Pen	Patch
Pipe	Gum		Cream
Water Pipe	Drink		Other
Blunt	Edibles		_____
Dabbed	Tincture		_____
	Oil		_____

Sweet
Fruity   Floral

Sour   Spicy

Earthy   Herbal
        Woodsy

Effects	Strength				
Peaceful	○	○	○	○	○
Sleepy	○	○	○	○	○
Pain Relief	○	○	○	○	○
Hungry	○	○	○	○	○
Uplifted	○	○	○	○	○
Creative	○	○	○	○	○

Try Again   ☐ Yes   ☐ No

Rating 🍁 🍁 🍁 🍁 🍁

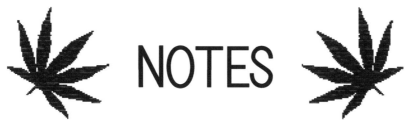

NOTES

STRAIN

Grower _____ Date _____

Acquired _____ $ _____

| THC Amount _____ | CBD Oil Amount _____ | ☐ Indica | ☐ Hybrid | ☐ Sativa |

☐ Flower ☐ Edible ☐ Concentrate

Symptoms Relieved

_____

_____

_____

_____

Consumed Method

Smoke	Ate	Vape	External
Rolled	Butter	Pen	Patch
Pipe	Gum		Cream
Water Pipe	Drink		Other
Blunt	Edibles		_____
Dabbed	Tincture		_____
	Oil		_____

Try Again ☐ Yes ☐ No

Sweet
Fruity   Floral
Sour   Spicy
Earthy   Herbal
Woodsy

Effects	Strength				
Peaceful	○	○	○	○	○
Sleepy	○	○	○	○	○
Pain Relief	○	○	○	○	○
Hungry	○	○	○	○	○
Uplifted	○	○	○	○	○
Creative	○	○	○	○	○

Rating

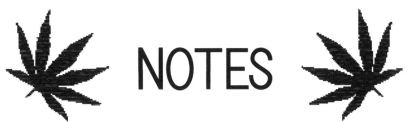

NOTES

STRAIN

Grower _____   Date _____

Acquired _____ $ _____

| THC Amount _____ | CBD Oil Amount _____ | ☐ Indica | ☐ Hybrid | ☐ Sativa |

☐ Flower   ☐ Edible   ☐ Concentrate

Symptoms Relieved

_____

_____

_____

_____

Consumed Method

Smoke	Ate	Vape	External
Rolled	Butter	Pen	Patch
Pipe	Gum		Cream
Water Pipe	Drink		Other
Blunt	Edibles		_____
Dabbed	Tincture		_____
	Oil		_____

Try Again   ☐ Yes   ☐ No

Sweet
Fruity   Floral
Sour   Spicy
Earthy   Herbal
Woodsy

Effects	Strength
Peaceful	○ ○ ○ ○ ○
Sleepy	○ ○ ○ ○ ○
Pain Relief	○ ○ ○ ○ ○
Hungry	○ ○ ○ ○ ○
Uplifted	○ ○ ○ ○ ○
Creative	○ ○ ○ ○ ○

Rating 🍁 🍁 🍁 🍁 🍁

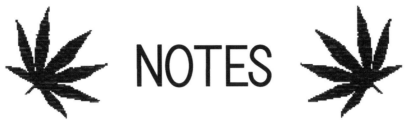

NOTES

STRAIN

Grower _____ Date _____

Acquired _____ $ _____

THC Amount _____   CBD Oil Amount _____   ☐ Indica   ☐ Hybrid   ☐ Sativa

☐ Flower   ☐ Edible   ☐ Concentrate

Symptoms Relieved

....

....

....

....

Sweet

Fruity   Floral

Sour   Spicy

Earthy   Herbal

Woodsy

Consumed Method

Smoke	Ate	Vape	External
Rolled	Butter	Pen	Patch
Pipe	Gum		Cream
Water Pipe	Drink		Other
Blunt	Edibles		_____
Dabbed	Tincture		_____
	Oil		_____

Effects	Strength				
Peaceful	○	○	○	○	○
Sleepy	○	○	○	○	○
Pain Relief	○	○	○	○	○
Hungry	○	○	○	○	○
Uplifted	○	○	○	○	○
Creative	○	○	○	○	○

Try Again   ☐ Yes   ☐ No

Rating   🌿 🌿 🌿 🌿 🌿

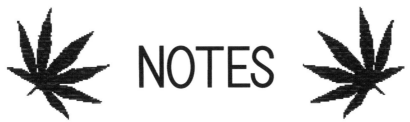

NOTES

STRAIN

Grower _____ Date _____

Acquired _____ $ _____

THC Amount _____ CBD Oil Amount _____ ☐ Indica ☐ Hybrid ☐ Sativa

☐ Flower ☐ Edible ☐ Concentrate

Symptoms Relieved

_____

_____

_____

_____

Sweet
Fruity   Floral
Sour   Spicy
Earthy   Herbal
Woodsy

Consumed Method

Smoke	Ate	Vape	External
Rolled	Butter	Pen	Patch
Pipe	Gum		Cream
Water Pipe	Drink		Other
Blunt	Edibles		_____
Dabbed	Tincture		_____
	Oil		_____

Effects	Strength				
Peaceful	◯	◯	◯	◯	◯
Sleepy	◯	◯	◯	◯	◯
Pain Relief	◯	◯	◯	◯	◯
Hungry	◯	◯	◯	◯	◯
Uplifted	◯	◯	◯	◯	◯
Creative	◯	◯	◯	◯	◯

Try Again ☐ Yes ☐ No

Rating 🌿 🌿 🌿 🌿 🌿

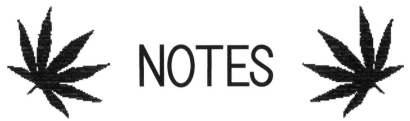

NOTES

STRAIN

Grower _____   Date _____

Acquired _____ $ _____

| THC Amount _____ | CBD Oil Amount _____ | ☐ Indica | ☐ Hybrid | ☐ Sativa |

☐ Flower   ☐ Edible   ☐ Concentrate

Symptoms Relieved

_____

_____

_____

_____

Consumed Method

Smoke	Ate	Vape	External
Rolled	Butter	Pen	Patch
Pipe	Gum		Cream
Water Pipe	Drink		Other
Blunt	Edibles		_____
Dabbed	Tincture		_____
	Oil		_____

Try Again   ☐ Yes   ☐ No

Sweet
Fruity
Floral
Sour
Spicy
Earthy
Herbal
Woodsy

Effects	Strength				
Peaceful	○	○	○	○	○
Sleepy	○	○	○	○	○
Pain Relief	○	○	○	○	○
Hungry	○	○	○	○	○
Uplifted	○	○	○	○	○
Creative	○	○	○	○	○

Rating 🍁 🍁 🍁 🍁 🍁

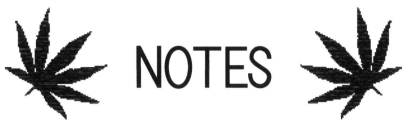

NOTES

STRAIN

Grower _____ Date _____

Acquired _____ $ _____

THC Amount _____ CBD Oil Amount _____ ☐ Indica ☐ Hybrid ☐ Sativa

☐ Flower ☐ Edible ☐ Concentrate

Symptoms Relieved

_____

_____

_____

_____

Sweet
Fruity   Floral
Sour   Spicy
Earthy   Herbal
Woodsy

Consumed Method

Smoke	Ate	Vape	External
Rolled	Butter	Pen	Patch
Pipe	Gum		Cream
Water Pipe	Drink		Other
Blunt	Edibles		_____
Dabbed	Tincture		_____
	Oil		_____

Effects	Strength				
Peaceful	○	○	○	○	○
Sleepy	○	○	○	○	○
Pain Relief	○	○	○	○	○
Hungry	○	○	○	○	○
Uplifted	○	○	○	○	○
Creative	○	○	○	○	○

Try Again ☐ Yes ☐ No

Rating

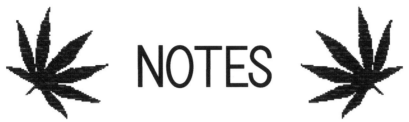

NOTES

STRAIN

Grower _____   Date _____

Acquired _____ $ _____

| THC Amount _____ | CBD Oil Amount _____ | ☐ Indica | ☐ Hybrid | ☐ Sativa |

☐ Flower   ☐ Edible   ☐ Concentrate

Symptoms Relieved

_____

_____

_____

_____

Consumed Method

Smoke	Ate	Vape	External
Rolled	Butter	Pen	Patch
Pipe	Gum		Cream
Water Pipe	Drink		Other
Blunt	Edibles		_____
Dabbed	Tincture		_____
	Oil		_____

Try Again   ☐ Yes   ☐ No

Sweet
Fruity   Floral

Sour   Spicy

Earthy   Herbal
Woodsy

Effects	Strength				
Peaceful	○	○	○	○	○
Sleepy	○	○	○	○	○
Pain Relief	○	○	○	○	○
Hungry	○	○	○	○	○
Uplifted	○	○	○	○	○
Creative	○	○	○	○	○

Rating 🍁 🍁 🍁 🍁 🍁

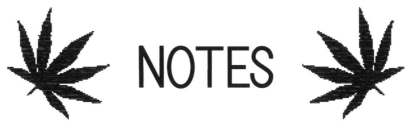

NOTES

STRAIN

Grower _____ Date _____

Acquired _____ $ _____

| THC Amount _____ | CBD Oil Amount _____ | ☐ Indica | ☐ Hybrid | ☐ Sativa |

☐ Flower   ☐ Edible   ☐ Concentrate

Symptoms Relieved

_____
_____
_____
_____

Sweet
Fruity   Floral
Sour   Spicy
Earthy   Herbal
Woodsy

Consumed Method

Smoke	Ate	Vape	External
Rolled	Butter	Pen	Patch
Pipe	Gum		Cream
Water Pipe	Drink		Other
Blunt	Edibles		_____
Dabbed	Tincture		_____
	Oil		_____

Effects	Strength				
Peaceful	○	○	○	○	○
Sleepy	○	○	○	○	○
Pain Relief	○	○	○	○	○
Hungry	○	○	○	○	○
Uplifted	○	○	○	○	○
Creative	○	○	○	○	○

Try Again   ☐ Yes   ☐ No

Rating 🍁 🍁 🍁 🍁 🍁

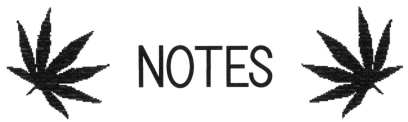

NOTES

STRAIN

Grower _____ Date _____

Acquired _____ $ _____

| THC Amount _____ | CBD Oil Amount _____ | ☐ Indica | ☐ Hybrid | ☐ Sativa |

☐ Flower   ☐ Edible   ☐ Concentrate

Symptoms Relieved

_____

_____

_____

_____

Consumed Method

Smoke	Ate	Vape	External
Rolled	Butter	Pen	Patch
Pipe	Gum		Cream
Water Pipe	Drink		Other
Blunt	Edibles		_____
Dabbed	Tincture		_____
	Oil		_____

Try Again   ☐ Yes   ☐ No

Flavor Wheel

Sweet, Fruity, Floral, Sour, Spicy, Earthy, Herbal, Woodsy

Effects — Strength

Effects	Strength				
Peaceful	○	○	○	○	○
Sleepy	○	○	○	○	○
Pain Relief	○	○	○	○	○
Hungry	○	○	○	○	○
Uplifted	○	○	○	○	○
Creative	○	○	○	○	○

Rating 🍁 🍁 🍁 🍁 🍁

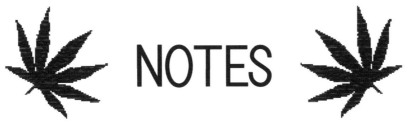

NOTES

STRAIN

Grower _____   Date _____

Acquired _____ $ _____

| THC Amount _____ | CBD Oil Amount _____ | ☐ Indica | ☐ Hybrid | ☐ Sativa |

☐ Flower   ☐ Edible   ☐ Concentrate

Symptoms Relieved

_____

_____

_____

_____

Sweet
Fruity   Floral
Sour   Spicy
Earthy   Herbal
Woodsy

Consumed Method

Smoke	Ate	Vape	External
Rolled	Butter	Pen	Patch
Pipe	Gum		Cream
Water Pipe	Drink		Other
Blunt	Edibles		_____
Dabbed	Tincture		_____
	Oil		_____

Effects	Strength				
Peaceful	○	○	○	○	○
Sleepy	○	○	○	○	○
Pain Relief	○	○	○	○	○
Hungry	○	○	○	○	○
Uplifted	○	○	○	○	○
Creative	○	○	○	○	○

Try Again   ☐ Yes   ☐ No

Rating 🌿 🌿 🌿 🌿 🌿

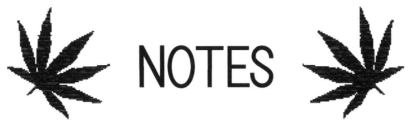

NOTES

STRAIN

Grower _____ Date _____

Acquired _____ $ _____

| THC Amount _____ | CBD Oil Amount _____ | ☐ Indica | ☐ Hybrid | ☐ Sativa |

☐ Flower   ☐ Edible   ☐ Concentrate

Symptoms Relieved

_____

_____

_____

_____

Consumed Method

Smoke	Ate	Vape	External
Rolled	Butter	Pen	Patch
Pipe	Gum		Cream
Water Pipe	Drink		Other
Blunt	Edibles		_____
Dabbed	Tincture		_____
	Oil		_____

Try Again   ☐ Yes   ☐ No

Flavor Wheel

Sweet
Fruity
Floral
Sour
Spicy
Earthy
Herbal
Woodsy

Effects	Strength				
Peaceful	○	○	○	○	○
Sleepy	○	○	○	○	○
Pain Relief	○	○	○	○	○
Hungry	○	○	○	○	○
Uplifted	○	○	○	○	○
Creative	○	○	○	○	○

Rating 🌿 🌿 🌿 🌿 🌿

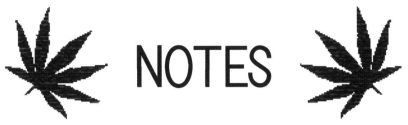

NOTES

STRAIN

Grower _____   Date _____

Acquired _____ $ _____

| THC Amount _____ | CBD Oil Amount _____ | ☐ Indica | ☐ Hybrid | ☐ Sativa |

☐ Flower   ☐ Edible   ☐ Concentrate

Symptoms Relieved

_____

_____

_____

_____

Sweet
Fruity   Floral

Sour   Spicy

Earthy   Herbal
Woodsy

Consumed Method

Smoke	Ate	Vape	External
Rolled	Butter	Pen	Patch
Pipe	Gum		Cream
Water Pipe	Drink		Other
Blunt	Edibles		_____
Dabbed	Tincture		_____
	Oil		_____

Effects	Strength				
Peaceful	○	○	○	○	○
Sleepy	○	○	○	○	○
Pain Relief	○	○	○	○	○
Hungry	○	○	○	○	○
Uplifted	○	○	○	○	○
Creative	○	○	○	○	○

Try Again   ☐ Yes   ☐ No

Rating 🍁 🍁 🍁 🍁 🍁

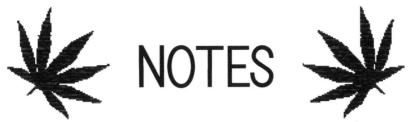

NOTES

STRAIN

Grower _____   Date _____

Acquired _____ $ _____

| THC Amount _____ | CBD Oil Amount _____ | ☐ Indica | ☐ Hybrid | ☐ Sativa |

☐ Flower   ☐ Edible   ☐ Concentrate

Symptoms Relieved

_____

_____

_____

_____

Sweet · Fruity · Floral · Sour · Spicy · Earthy · Herbal · Woodsy

Consumed Method

Smoke	Ate	Vape	External
Rolled	Butter	Pen	Patch
Pipe	Gum		Cream
Water Pipe	Drink		Other
Blunt	Edibles		_____
Dabbed	Tincture		_____
	Oil		_____

Effects	Strength				
Peaceful	○	○	○	○	○
Sleepy	○	○	○	○	○
Pain Relief	○	○	○	○	○
Hungry	○	○	○	○	○
Uplifted	○	○	○	○	○
Creative	○	○	○	○	○

Try Again   ☐ Yes   ☐ No

Rating

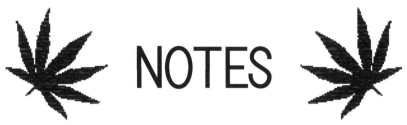

NOTES

STRAIN

Grower _____ Date _____

Acquired _____ $ _____

| THC Amount _____ CBD Oil Amount _____ | ☐ Indica | ☐ Hybrid | ☐ Sativa |

☐ Flower   ☐ Edible   ☐ Concentrate

Symptoms Relieved

_____

_____

_____

_____

Consumed Method

Smoke	Ate	Vape	External
Rolled	Butter	Pen	Patch
Pipe	Gum		Cream
Water Pipe	Drink		Other
Blunt	Edibles		_____
Dabbed	Tincture		_____
	Oil		_____

Try Again ☐ Yes   ☐ No

Sweet

Fruity

Floral

Sour

Spicy

Earthy

Herbal

Woodsy

Effects	Strength				
Peaceful	○	○	○	○	○
Sleepy	○	○	○	○	○
Pain Relief	○	○	○	○	○
Hungry	○	○	○	○	○
Uplifted	○	○	○	○	○
Creative	○	○	○	○	○

Rating

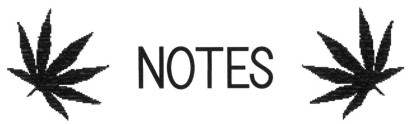

NOTES

STRAIN

Grower _____   Date _____

Acquired _____ $ _____

| THC Amount _____ | CBD Oil Amount _____ | ☐ Indica | ☐ Hybrid | ☐ Sativa |

☐ Flower   ☐ Edible   ☐ Concentrate

Symptoms Relieved

_____

_____

_____

_____

Sweet
Fruity   Floral

Sour   Spicy

Earthy   Herbal
Woodsy

Consumed Method

Smoke	Ate	Vape	External
Rolled	Butter	Pen	Patch
Pipe	Gum		Cream
Water Pipe	Drink		Other
Blunt	Edibles		_____
Dabbed	Tincture		_____
	Oil		_____

Effects	Strength				
Peaceful	○	○	○	○	○
Sleepy	○	○	○	○	○
Pain Relief	○	○	○	○	○
Hungry	○	○	○	○	○
Uplifted	○	○	○	○	○
Creative	○	○	○	○	○

Try Again   ☐ Yes   ☐ No

Rating

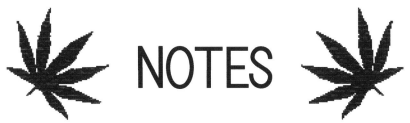

NOTES

STRAIN

Grower _____ Date _____

Acquired _____ $ _____

THC Amount _____ CBD Oil Amount _____ ☐ Indica ☐ Hybrid ☐ Sativa

☐ Flower ☐ Edible ☐ Concentrate

Symptoms Relieved

_____

_____

_____

_____

Consumed Method

Smoke	Ate	Vape	External
Rolled	Butter	Pen	Patch
Pipe	Gum		Cream
Water Pipe	Drink		Other
Blunt	Edibles		_____
Dabbed	Tincture		_____
	Oil		_____

Try Again ☐ Yes ☐ No

Sweet

Fruity   Floral

Sour   Spicy

Earthy   Herbal

Woodsy

Effects	Strength
Peaceful	○ ○ ○ ○ ○
Sleepy	○ ○ ○ ○ ○
Pain Relief	○ ○ ○ ○ ○
Hungry	○ ○ ○ ○ ○
Uplifted	○ ○ ○ ○ ○
Creative	○ ○ ○ ○ ○

Rating 🍁 🍁 🍁 🍁 🍁

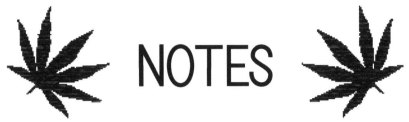

NOTES

STRAIN

Grower _____   Date _____

Acquired _____ $ _____

| THC Amount _____   CBD Oil Amount _____ | ☐ Indica | ☐ Hybrid | ☐ Sativa |

☐ Flower   ☐ Edible   ☐ Concentrate

Symptoms Relieved

_____

_____

_____

_____

Sweet

Fruity   Floral

Sour   Spicy

Earthy   Herbal

Woodsy

Consumed Method

Smoke	Ate	Vape	External
Rolled	Butter	Pen	Patch
Pipe	Gum		Cream
Water Pipe	Drink		Other
Blunt	Edibles		_____
Dabbed	Tincture		_____
	Oil		_____

Effects   Strength

Peaceful	○ ○ ○ ○ ○
Sleepy	○ ○ ○ ○ ○
Pain Relief	○ ○ ○ ○ ○
Hungry	○ ○ ○ ○ ○
Uplifted	○ ○ ○ ○ ○
Creative	○ ○ ○ ○ ○

Try Again   ☐ Yes   ☐ No

Rating 🌿 🌿 🌿 🌿 🌿

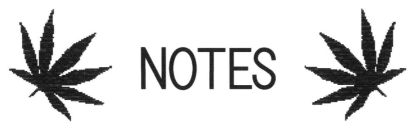

NOTES

STRAIN

Grower _____   Date _____

Acquired _____ $ _____

| THC Amount _____ | CBD Oil Amount _____ | ☐ Indica | ☐ Hybrid | ☐ Sativa |

☐ Flower   ☐ Edible   ☐ Concentrate

Symptoms Relieved

_____

_____

_____

_____

Consumed Method

Smoke	Ate	Vape	External
Rolled	Butter	Pen	Patch
Pipe	Gum		Cream
Water Pipe	Drink		Other
Blunt	Edibles		_____
Dabbed	Tincture		_____
	Oil		_____

Try Again   ☐ Yes   ☐ No

Sweet
Fruity
Floral
Sour
Spicy
Earthy
Herbal
Woodsy

Effects	Strength				
Peaceful	○	○	○	○	○
Sleepy	○	○	○	○	○
Pain Relief	○	○	○	○	○
Hungry	○	○	○	○	○
Uplifted	○	○	○	○	○
Creative	○	○	○	○	○

Rating 🌿 🌿 🌿 🌿 🌿

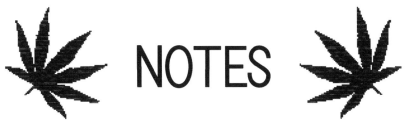

NOTES

STRAIN

Grower _____ Date _____

Acquired _____ $ _____

| THC Amount _____ CBD Oil Amount _____ | ☐ Indica | ☐ Hybrid | ☐ Sativa |

☐ Flower   ☐ Edible   ☐ Concentrate

Symptoms Relieved

_____

_____

_____

_____

Consumed Method

Smoke	Ate	Vape	External
Rolled	Butter	Pen	Patch
Pipe	Gum		Cream
Water Pipe	Drink		Other
Blunt	Edibles		_____
Dabbed	Tincture		_____
	Oil		_____

Try Again   ☐ Yes   ☐ No

Sweet
Fruity   Floral
Sour   Spicy
Earthy   Herbal
Woodsy

Effects	Strength				
Peaceful	○	○	○	○	○
Sleepy	○	○	○	○	○
Pain Relief	○	○	○	○	○
Hungry	○	○	○	○	○
Uplifted	○	○	○	○	○
Creative	○	○	○	○	○

Rating 🌿 🌿 🌿 🌿 🌿

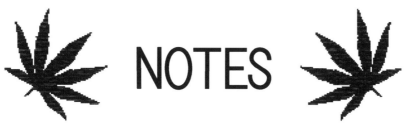

NOTES

STRAIN

Grower _____ Date _____

Acquired _____ $ _____

| THC Amount _____ CBD Oil Amount _____ | ☐ Indica | ☐ Hybrid | ☐ Sativa |

☐ Flower   ☐ Edible   ☐ Concentrate

Symptoms Relieved

_____

_____

_____

_____

Consumed Method

Smoke	Ate	Vape	External
Rolled	Butter	Pen	Patch
Pipe	Gum		Cream
Water Pipe	Drink		Other
Blunt	Edibles		_____
Dabbed	Tincture		_____
	Oil		_____

Try Again ☐ Yes   ☐ No

Sweet
Fruity
Floral
Sour
Spicy
Earthy
Herbal
Woodsy

Effects	Strength				
Peaceful	○	○	○	○	○
Sleepy	○	○	○	○	○
Pain Relief	○	○	○	○	○
Hungry	○	○	○	○	○
Uplifted	○	○	○	○	○
Creative	○	○	○	○	○

Rating 🌿 🌿 🌿 🌿 🌿

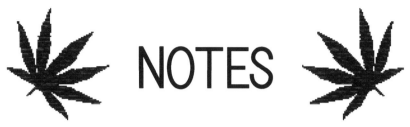

NOTES

STRAIN

Grower _____   Date _____

Acquired _____ $ _____

| THC Amount _____ CBD Oil Amount _____ | ☐ Indica | ☐ Hybrid | ☐ Sativa |

☐ Flower   ☐ Edible   ☐ Concentrate

Symptoms Relieved

_____

_____

_____

_____

Consumed Method

Smoke	Ate	Vape	External
Rolled	Butter	Pen	Patch
Pipe	Gum		Cream
Water Pipe	Drink		Other
Blunt	Edibles		_____
Dabbed	Tincture		_____
	Oil		_____

Try Again   ☐ Yes   ☐ No

Sweet

Fruity   Floral

Sour   Spicy

Earthy   Herbal

Woodsy

Effects	Strength
Peaceful	○ ○ ○ ○ ○
Sleepy	○ ○ ○ ○ ○
Pain Relief	○ ○ ○ ○ ○
Hungry	○ ○ ○ ○ ○
Uplifted	○ ○ ○ ○ ○
Creative	○ ○ ○ ○ ○

Rating 🌿 🌿 🌿 🌿 🌿

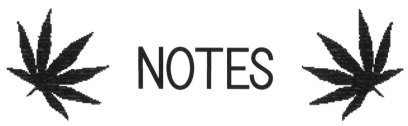

NOTES

STRAIN

Grower _____   Date _____

Acquired _____ $ _____

THC Amount _____ CBD Oil Amount _____	☐ Indica	☐ Hybrid	☐ Sativa

☐ Flower   ☐ Edible   ☐ Concentrate

Symptoms Relieved

_____

_____

_____

Consumed Method

Smoke	Ate	Vape	External
Rolled	Butter	Pen	Patch
Pipe	Gum		Cream
Water Pipe	Drink		Other
Blunt	Edibles		_____
Dabbed	Tincture		_____
	Oil		_____

Try Again   ☐ Yes   ☐ No

Sweet
Fruity   Floral
Sour   Spicy
Earthy   Herbal
Woodsy

Effects	Strength				
Peaceful	○	○	○	○	○
Sleepy	○	○	○	○	○
Pain Relief	○	○	○	○	○
Hungry	○	○	○	○	○
Uplifted	○	○	○	○	○
Creative	○	○	○	○	○

Rating 🍁 🍁 🍁 🍁 🍁

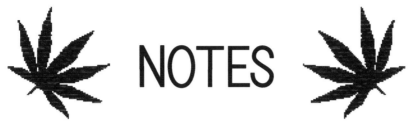

NOTES

STRAIN

Grower _____ Date _____

Acquired _____ $ _____

| THC Amount _____ CBD Oil Amount _____ | ☐ Indica | ☐ Hybrid | ☐ Sativa |

☐ Flower   ☐ Edible   ☐ Concentrate

Symptoms Relieved

_____
_____
_____
_____

Sweet

Fruity   Floral

Sour   Spicy

Earthy   Herbal

Woodsy

Consumed Method

Smoke	Ate	Vape	External
Rolled	Butter	Pen	Patch
Pipe	Gum		Cream
Water Pipe	Drink		Other
Blunt	Edibles		_____
Dabbed	Tincture		_____
	Oil		_____

Effects	Strength				
Peaceful	○	○	○	○	○
Sleepy	○	○	○	○	○
Pain Relief	○	○	○	○	○
Hungry	○	○	○	○	○
Uplifted	○	○	○	○	○
Creative	○	○	○	○	○

Try Again   ☐ Yes   ☐ No

Rating

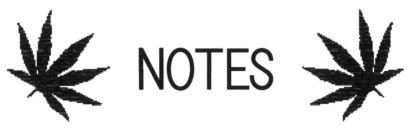

NOTES

STRAIN

Grower _____   Date _____

Acquired _____ $ _____

| THC Amount _____ | CBD Oil Amount _____ | ☐ Indica | ☐ Hybrid | ☐ Sativa |

☐ Flower   ☐ Edible   ☐ Concentrate

Symptoms Relieved

_____

_____

_____

_____

Consumed Method

Smoke	Ate	Vape	External
Rolled	Butter	Pen	Patch
Pipe	Gum		Cream
Water Pipe	Drink		Other
Blunt	Edibles		_____
Dabbed	Tincture		_____
	Oil		_____

Try Again ☐ Yes ☐ No

Sweet

Fruity

Floral

Sour

Spicy

Earthy

Herbal

Woodsy

Effects	Strength				
Peaceful	○	○	○	○	○
Sleepy	○	○	○	○	○
Pain Relief	○	○	○	○	○
Hungry	○	○	○	○	○
Uplifted	○	○	○	○	○
Creative	○	○	○	○	○

Rating 🍁 🍁 🍁 🍁 🍁

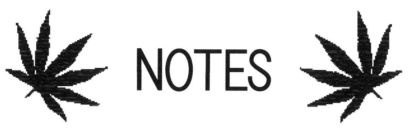

NOTES

STRAIN

Grower _____   Date _____

Acquired _____ $ _____

THC Amount _____	CBD Oil Amount _____	☐ Indica	☐ Hybrid	☐ Sativa

☐ Flower   ☐ Edible   ☐ Concentrate

Symptoms Relieved

_____

_____

_____

_____

Sweet
Fruity   Floral

Sour   Spicy

Earthy   Herbal
Woodsy

Consumed Method

Smoke	Ate	Vape	External
Rolled	Butter	Pen	Patch
Pipe	Gum		Cream
Water Pipe	Drink		Other
Blunt	Edibles		_____
Dabbed	Tincture		_____
	Oil		_____

Effects	Strength				
Peaceful	○	○	○	○	○
Sleepy	○	○	○	○	○
Pain Relief	○	○	○	○	○
Hungry	○	○	○	○	○
Uplifted	○	○	○	○	○
Creative	○	○	○	○	○

Try Again   ☐ Yes   ☐ No

Rating

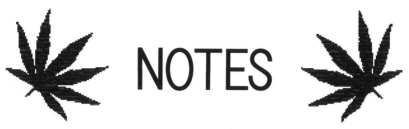

NOTES

STRAIN

Grower _____ Date _____

Acquired _____ $ _____

| THC Amount _____ | CBD Oil Amount _____ | ☐ Indica | ☐ Hybrid | ☐ Sativa |

☐ Flower ☐ Edible ☐ Concentrate

Symptoms Relieved

_____

_____

_____

_____

Sweet

Fruity   Floral

Sour   ●   Spicy

Earthy   Herbal

Woodsy

Consumed Method

Smoke	Ate	Vape	External
Rolled	Butter	Pen	Patch
Pipe	Gum		Cream
Water Pipe	Drink		Other
Blunt	Edibles		_____
Dabbed	Tincture		_____
	Oil		_____

Effects	Strength				
Peaceful	◯	◯	◯	◯	◯
Sleepy	◯	◯	◯	◯	◯
Pain Relief	◯	◯	◯	◯	◯
Hungry	◯	◯	◯	◯	◯
Uplifted	◯	◯	◯	◯	◯
Creative	◯	◯	◯	◯	◯

Try Again ☐ Yes ☐ No

Rating 🌿 🌿 🌿 🌿 🌿

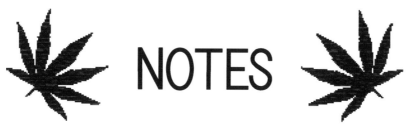

NOTES

STRAIN

Grower _____ Date _____

Acquired _____ $ _____

| THC Amount _____ | CBD Oil Amount _____ | ☐ Indica | ☐ Hybrid | ☐ Sativa |

☐ Flower   ☐ Edible   ☐ Concentrate

Symptoms Relieved

_____

_____

_____

_____

Consumed Method

Smoke	Ate	Vape	External
Rolled	Butter	Pen	Patch
Pipe	Gum		Cream
Water Pipe	Drink		Other
Blunt	Edibles		_____
Dabbed	Tincture		_____
	Oil		_____

Try Again   ☐ Yes   ☐ No

Aroma Wheel

Sweet
Fruity
Floral
Sour
Spicy
Earthy
Herbal
Woodsy

Effects	Strength				
Peaceful	◯	◯	◯	◯	◯
Sleepy	◯	◯	◯	◯	◯
Pain Relief	◯	◯	◯	◯	◯
Hungry	◯	◯	◯	◯	◯
Uplifted	◯	◯	◯	◯	◯
Creative	◯	◯	◯	◯	◯

Rating 🌿 🌿 🌿 🌿 🌿

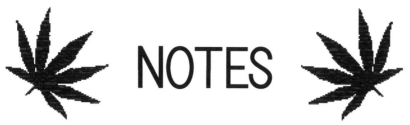

NOTES

STRAIN

Grower _____   Date _____

Acquired _____ $ _____

| THC Amount _____ | CBD Oil Amount _____ | ☐ Indica | ☐ Hybrid | ☐ Sativa |

☐ Flower   ☐ Edible   ☐ Concentrate

Symptoms Relieved

_____

_____

_____

_____

Sweet

Fruity

Floral

Sour

Spicy

Earthy

Herbal

Woodsy

Consumed Method

Smoke	Ate	Vape	External
Rolled	Butter	Pen	Patch
Pipe	Gum		Cream
Water Pipe	Drink		Other
Blunt	Edibles		_____
Dabbed	Tincture		_____
	Oil		_____

Effects	Strength				
Peaceful	○	○	○	○	○
Sleepy	○	○	○	○	○
Pain Relief	○	○	○	○	○
Hungry	○	○	○	○	○
Uplifted	○	○	○	○	○
Creative	○	○	○	○	○

Try Again   ☐ Yes   ☐ No

Rating

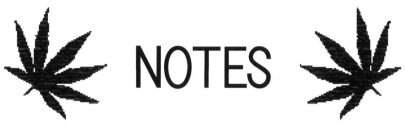

NOTES

STRAIN

Grower _____ Date _____

Acquired _____ $ _____

THC Amount _____ CBD Oil Amount _____ ☐ Indica ☐ Hybrid ☐ Sativa

☐ Flower ☐ Edible ☐ Concentrate

Symptoms Relieved

_____
_____
_____
_____

Sweet

Fruity   Floral

Sour   Spicy

Earthy   Herbal

Woodsy

Consumed Method

Smoke	Ate	Vape	External
Rolled	Butter	Pen	Patch
Pipe	Gum		Cream
Water Pipe	Drink		Other
Blunt	Edibles		_____
Dabbed	Tincture		_____
	Oil		_____

Effects	Strength				
Peaceful	○	○	○	○	○
Sleepy	○	○	○	○	○
Pain Relief	○	○	○	○	○
Hungry	○	○	○	○	○
Uplifted	○	○	○	○	○
Creative	○	○	○	○	○

Try Again ☐ Yes ☐ No

Rating 🍁 🍁 🍁 🍁 🍁

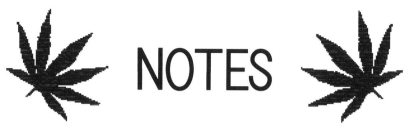

NOTES

STRAIN

Grower _____   Date _____

Acquired _____ $ _____

THC Amount _____	CBD Oil Amount _____	☐ Indica	☐ Hybrid	☐ Sativa

☐ Flower   ☐ Edible   ☐ Concentrate

Symptoms Relieved

_____

_____

_____

_____

Sweet

Fruity   Floral

Sour   Spicy

Earthy   Herbal

Woodsy

Consumed Method

Smoke	Ate	Vape	External
Rolled	Butter	Pen	Patch
Pipe	Gum		Cream
Water Pipe	Drink		Other
Blunt	Edibles		_____
Dabbed	Tincture		_____
	Oil		_____

Effects	Strength				
Peaceful	◯	◯	◯	◯	◯
Sleepy	◯	◯	◯	◯	◯
Pain Relief	◯	◯	◯	◯	◯
Hungry	◯	◯	◯	◯	◯
Uplifted	◯	◯	◯	◯	◯
Creative	◯	◯	◯	◯	◯

Try Again   ☐ Yes   ☐ No

Rating

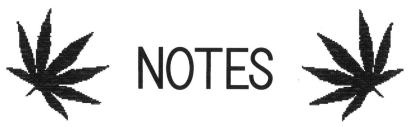

NOTES

STRAIN _____

Grower _____   Date _____

Acquired _____ $ _____

| THC Amount _____ | CBD Oil Amount _____ | ☐ Indica | ☐ Hybrid | ☐ Sativa |

☐ Flower   ☐ Edible   ☐ Concentrate

Symptoms Relieved

_____

_____

_____

_____

Sweet
Fruity   Floral

Sour   Spicy

Earthy   Herbal
Woodsy

Consumed Method

Smoke	Ate	Vape	External
Rolled	Butter	Pen	Patch
Pipe	Gum		Cream
Water Pipe	Drink		Other
Blunt	Edibles		_____
Dabbed	Tincture		_____
	Oil		_____

Effects	Strength				
Peaceful	○	○	○	○	○
Sleepy	○	○	○	○	○
Pain Relief	○	○	○	○	○
Hungry	○	○	○	○	○
Uplifted	○	○	○	○	○
Creative	○	○	○	○	○

Try Again   ☐ Yes   ☐ No

Rating   🍁 🍁 🍁 🍁 🍁

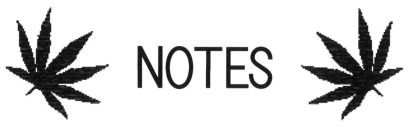

NOTES

STRAIN

Grower _____ Date _____

Acquired _____ $ _____

| THC Amount _____ | CBD Oil Amount _____ | ☐ Indica | ☐ Hybrid | ☐ Sativa |

☐ Flower   ☐ Edible   ☐ Concentrate

Symptoms Relieved

_____

_____

_____

_____

Sweet

Fruity   Floral

Sour   Spicy

Earthy   Herbal

Woodsy

Consumed Method

Smoke	Ate	Vape	External
Rolled	Butter	Pen	Patch
Pipe	Gum		Cream
Water Pipe	Drink		Other
Blunt	Edibles		_____
Dabbed	Tincture		_____
	Oil		_____

Effects	Strength				
Peaceful	○	○	○	○	○
Sleepy	○	○	○	○	○
Pain Relief	○	○	○	○	○
Hungry	○	○	○	○	○
Uplifted	○	○	○	○	○
Creative	○	○	○	○	○

Try Again   ☐ Yes   ☐ No

Rating   🍁 🍁 🍁 🍁 🍁

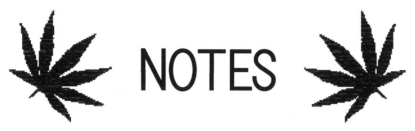

NOTES

STRAIN

Grower _____ Date _____

Acquired _____ $ _____

| THC Amount _____ | CBD Oil Amount _____ | ☐ Indica | ☐ Hybrid | ☐ Sativa |

☐ Flower   ☐ Edible   ☐ Concentrate

Symptoms Relieved

_____
_____
_____
_____

Sweet

Fruity   Floral

Sour   Spicy

Earthy   Herbal

Woodsy

Consumed Method

Smoke	Ate	Vape	External
Rolled	Butter	Pen	Patch
Pipe	Gum		Cream
Water Pipe	Drink		Other
Blunt	Edibles		_____
Dabbed	Tincture		_____
	Oil		_____

Effects	Strength
Peaceful	○ ○ ○ ○ ○
Sleepy	○ ○ ○ ○ ○
Pain Relief	○ ○ ○ ○ ○
Hungry	○ ○ ○ ○ ○
Uplifted	○ ○ ○ ○ ○
Creative	○ ○ ○ ○ ○

Try Again   ☐ Yes   ☐ No

Rating 🌿 🌿 🌿 🌿 🌿

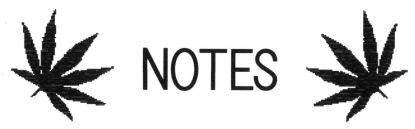

NOTES

STRAIN

Grower _____ Date _____

Acquired _____ $ _____

| THC Amount _____ | CBD Oil Amount _____ | ☐ Indica | ☐ Hybrid | ☐ Sativa |

☐ Flower   ☐ Edible   ☐ Concentrate

Symptoms Relieved

_____

_____

_____

_____

Sweet

Fruity   Floral

Sour   Spicy

Earthy   Herbal

Woodsy

Consumed Method

Smoke	Ate	Vape	External
Rolled	Butter	Pen	Patch
Pipe	Gum		Cream
Water Pipe	Drink		Other
Blunt	Edibles		_____
Dabbed	Tincture		_____
	Oil		_____

Effects	Strength				
Peaceful	○	○	○	○	○
Sleepy	○	○	○	○	○
Pain Relief	○	○	○	○	○
Hungry	○	○	○	○	○
Uplifted	○	○	○	○	○
Creative	○	○	○	○	○

Try Again   ☐ Yes   ☐ No

Rating

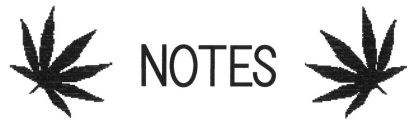

NOTES

STRAIN

Grower _____   Date _____

Acquired _____ $ _____

| THC Amount _____ | CBD Oil Amount _____ | ☐ Indica | ☐ Hybrid | ☐ Sativa |

☐ Flower   ☐ Edible   ☐ Concentrate

Symptoms Relieved

_____

_____

_____

_____

_____

Sweet
Fruity   Floral
Sour   Spicy
Earthy   Herbal
Woodsy

Consumed Method

Smoke	Ate	Vape	External
Rolled	Butter	Pen	Patch
Pipe	Gum		Cream
Water Pipe	Drink		Other
Blunt	Edibles		_____
Dabbed	Tincture		_____
	Oil		_____

Effects	Strength				
Peaceful	○	○	○	○	○
Sleepy	○	○	○	○	○
Pain Relief	○	○	○	○	○
Hungry	○	○	○	○	○
Uplifted	○	○	○	○	○
Creative	○	○	○	○	○

Try Again   ☐ Yes   ☐ No

Rating 🌿 🌿 🌿 🌿 🌿

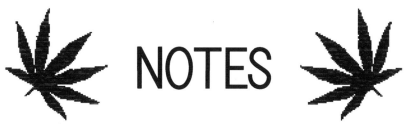

NOTES

STRAIN

Grower _____ Date _____

Acquired _____ $ _____

| THC Amount _____ | CBD Oil Amount _____ | ☐ Indica | ☐ Hybrid | ☐ Sativa |

☐ Flower ☐ Edible ☐ Concentrate

Symptoms Relieved

_____

_____

_____

_____

Sweet

Fruity   Floral

Sour   Spicy

Earthy   Herbal

Woodsy

Consumed Method

Smoke	Ate	Vape	External
Rolled	Butter	Pen	Patch
Pipe	Gum		Cream
Water Pipe	Drink		Other
Blunt	Edibles		_____
Dabbed	Tincture		_____
	Oil		_____

Effects	Strength				
Peaceful	◯	◯	◯	◯	◯
Sleepy	◯	◯	◯	◯	◯
Pain Relief	◯	◯	◯	◯	◯
Hungry	◯	◯	◯	◯	◯
Uplifted	◯	◯	◯	◯	◯
Creative	◯	◯	◯	◯	◯

Try Again ☐ Yes ☐ No

Rating 🌿 🌿 🌿 🌿 🌿

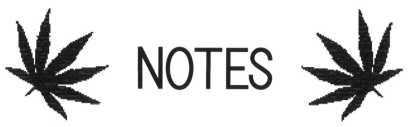

NOTES

STRAIN

Grower _____ Date _____

Acquired _____ $ _____

| THC Amount _____ | CBD Oil Amount _____ | ☐ Indica | ☐ Hybrid | ☐ Sativa |

☐ Flower ☐ Edible ☐ Concentrate

Symptoms Relieved

_____
_____
_____
_____
_____

Consumed Method

Smoke   Ate   Vape   External

Rolled   Butter   Pen   Patch

Pipe   Gum   Cream

Water Pipe Drink   Other

Blunt   Edibles   _____

Dabbed   Tincture   _____

           Oil   _____

Sweet

Fruity   Floral

Sour   Spicy

Earthy   Herbal

Woodsy

Effects — Strength

Effects	Strength				
Peaceful	○	○	○	○	○
Sleepy	○	○	○	○	○
Pain Relief	○	○	○	○	○
Hungry	○	○	○	○	○
Uplifted	○	○	○	○	○
Creative	○	○	○	○	○

Try Again ☐ Yes ☐ No

Rating

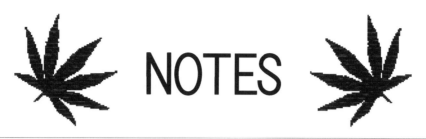

NOTES

STRAIN

Grower _____   Date _____

Acquired _____ $ _____

| THC Amount _____ | CBD Oil Amount _____ | ☐ Indica | ☐ Hybrid | ☐ Sativa |

☐ Flower   ☐ Edible   ☐ Concentrate

Symptoms Relieved

_____
_____
_____
_____

Sweet

Fruity   Floral

Sour   Spicy

Earthy   Herbal

Woodsy

Consumed Method

Smoke	Ate	Vape	External
Rolled	Butter	Pen	Patch
Pipe	Gum		Cream
Water Pipe	Drink		Other
Blunt	Edibles		_____
Dabbed	Tincture		_____
	Oil		_____

Effects	Strength				
Peaceful	○	○	○	○	○
Sleepy	○	○	○	○	○
Pain Relief	○	○	○	○	○
Hungry	○	○	○	○	○
Uplifted	○	○	○	○	○
Creative	○	○	○	○	○

Try Again   ☐ Yes   ☐ No

Rating 🌿 🌿 🌿 🌿 🌿

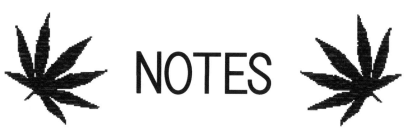# NOTES

STRAIN _____

Grower _____ Date _____

Acquired _____ $ _____

| THC Amount _____ | CBD Oil Amount _____ | ☐ Indica | ☐ Hybrid | ☐ Sativa |

☐ Flower   ☐ Edible   ☐ Concentrate

Symptoms Relieved

_____

_____

_____

_____

Consumed Method

Smoke	Ate	Vape	External
Rolled	Butter	Pen	Patch
Pipe	Gum		Cream
Water Pipe	Drink		Other
Blunt	Edibles		_____
Dabbed	Tincture		_____
	Oil		_____

Sweet
Fruity   Floral
Sour   Spicy
Earthy   Herbal
        Woodsy

Effects	Strength				
Peaceful	○	○	○	○	○
Sleepy	○	○	○	○	○
Pain Relief	○	○	○	○	○
Hungry	○	○	○	○	○
Uplifted	○	○	○	○	○
Creative	○	○	○	○	○

Try Again   ☐ Yes   ☐ No

Rating

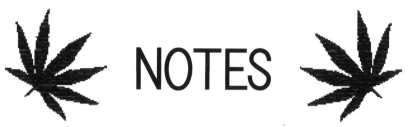

NOTES

STRAIN

Grower _____ Date _____

Acquired _____ $ _____

| THC Amount _____ CBD Oil Amount _____ | ☐ Indica | ☐ Hybrid | ☐ Sativa |

☐ Flower   ☐ Edible   ☐ Concentrate

Symptoms Relieved

_____

_____

_____

_____

Consumed Method

Smoke	Ate	Vape	External
Rolled	Butter	Pen	Patch
Pipe	Gum		Cream
Water Pipe	Drink		Other
Blunt	Edibles		_____
Dabbed	Tincture		_____
	Oil		_____

Try Again   ☐ Yes   ☐ No

Sweet

Fruity

Floral

Sour

Spicy

Earthy

Herbal

Woodsy

Effects	Strength				
Peaceful	◯	◯	◯	◯	◯
Sleepy	◯	◯	◯	◯	◯
Pain Relief	◯	◯	◯	◯	◯
Hungry	◯	◯	◯	◯	◯
Uplifted	◯	◯	◯	◯	◯
Creative	◯	◯	◯	◯	◯

Rating

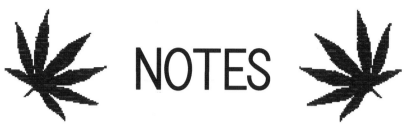

NOTES

STRAIN

Grower _____   Date _____

Acquired _____ $ _____

| THC Amount _____ | CBD Oil Amount _____ | ☐ Indica | ☐ Hybrid | ☐ Sativa |

☐ Flower   ☐ Edible   ☐ Concentrate

Symptoms Relieved

_____

_____

_____

_____

Sweet

Fruity   Floral

Sour   Spicy

Earthy   Herbal

Woodsy

Consumed Method

Smoke	Ate	Vape	External
Rolled	Butter	Pen	Patch
Pipe	Gum		Cream
Water Pipe	Drink		Other
Blunt	Edibles		_____
Dabbed	Tincture		_____
	Oil		_____

Effects	Strength				
Peaceful	○	○	○	○	○
Sleepy	○	○	○	○	○
Pain Relief	○	○	○	○	○
Hungry	○	○	○	○	○
Uplifted	○	○	○	○	○
Creative	○	○	○	○	○

Try Again ☐ Yes ☐ No

Rating 🌿 🌿 🌿 🌿 🌿

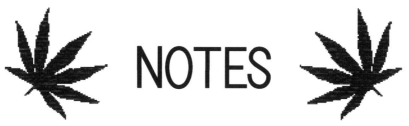

NOTES

STRAIN

Grower _____   Date _____

Acquired _____ $ _____

| THC Amount _____ | CBD Oil Amount _____ | ☐ Indica | ☐ Hybrid | ☐ Sativa |

☐ Flower   ☐ Edible   ☐ Concentrate

Symptoms Relieved

_____

_____

_____

_____

Sweet

Fruity   Floral

Sour   Spicy

Earthy   Herbal

Woodsy

Consumed Method

Smoke	Ate	Vape	External
Rolled	Butter	Pen	Patch
Pipe	Gum		Cream
Water Pipe	Drink		Other
Blunt	Edibles		_____
Dabbed	Tincture		_____
	Oil		_____

Effects	Strength				
Peaceful	○	○	○	○	○
Sleepy	○	○	○	○	○
Pain Relief	○	○	○	○	○
Hungry	○	○	○	○	○
Uplifted	○	○	○	○	○
Creative	○	○	○	○	○

Try Again   ☐ Yes   ☐ No

Rating   🍁 🍁 🍁 🍁 🍁

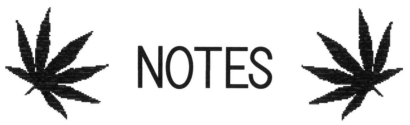

NOTES

STRAIN _____

Grower _____ Date _____

Acquired _____ $ _____

| THC Amount _____ | CBD Oil Amount _____ | ☐ Indica | ☐ Hybrid | ☐ Sativa |

☐ Flower   ☐ Edible   ☐ Concentrate

Symptoms Relieved

_____

_____

_____

_____

Sweet
Fruity   Floral
Sour   Spicy
Earthy   Herbal
Woodsy

Consumed Method

Smoke	Ate	Vape	External
Rolled	Butter	Pen	Patch
Pipe	Gum		Cream
Water Pipe	Drink		Other
Blunt	Edibles		_____
Dabbed	Tincture		_____
	Oil		_____

Effects — Strength

Effects	Strength				
Peaceful	○	○	○	○	○
Sleepy	○	○	○	○	○
Pain Relief	○	○	○	○	○
Hungry	○	○	○	○	○
Uplifted	○	○	○	○	○
Creative	○	○	○	○	○

Try Again   ☐ Yes   ☐ No

Rating 🌿 🌿 🌿 🌿 🌿

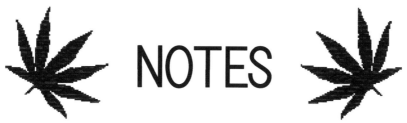

NOTES

STRAIN

Grower _____ Date _____

Acquired _____ $ _____

THC Amount _____ CBD Oil Amount _____ ☐ Indica ☐ Hybrid ☐ Sativa

☐ Flower ☐ Edible ☐ Concentrate

Symptoms Relieved

_____
_____
_____
_____

Sweet
Fruity   Floral

Sour   Spicy

Earthy   Herbal
Woodsy

Consumed Method

Smoke	Ate	Vape	External
Rolled	Butter	Pen	Patch
Pipe	Gum		Cream
Water Pipe	Drink		Other
Blunt	Edibles		_____
Dabbed	Tincture		_____
	Oil		_____

Effects	Strength				
Peaceful	○	○	○	○	○
Sleepy	○	○	○	○	○
Pain Relief	○	○	○	○	○
Hungry	○	○	○	○	○
Uplifted	○	○	○	○	○
Creative	○	○	○	○	○

Try Again   ☐ Yes   ☐ No

Rating

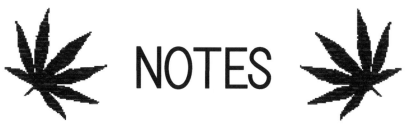

NOTES

STRAIN

Grower _____   Date _____

Acquired _____ $ _____

| THC Amount _____ | CBD Oil Amount _____ | ☐ Indica | ☐ Hybrid | ☐ Sativa |

☐ Flower   ☐ Edible   ☐ Concentrate

Symptoms Relieved

_____

_____

_____

Consumed Method

Smoke	Ate	Vape	External
Rolled	Butter	Pen	Patch
Pipe	Gum		Cream
Water Pipe	Drink		Other
Blunt	Edibles		_____
Dabbed	Tincture		_____
	Oil		_____

Try Again   ☐ Yes   ☐ No

Sweet
Fruity   Floral

Sour   Spicy

Earthy   Herbal
Woodsy

Effects	Strength				
Peaceful	○	○	○	○	○
Sleepy	○	○	○	○	○
Pain Relief	○	○	○	○	○
Hungry	○	○	○	○	○
Uplifted	○	○	○	○	○
Creative	○	○	○	○	○

Rating   🍁 🍁 🍁 🍁 🍁

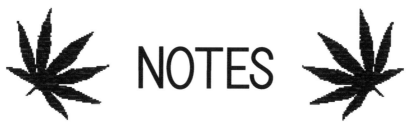

NOTES

STRAIN

Grower _____ Date _____

Acquired _____ $ _____

| THC Amount _____ | CBD Oil Amount _____ | ☐ Indica | ☐ Hybrid | ☐ Sativa |

☐ Flower   ☐ Edible   ☐ Concentrate

Symptoms Relieved

_____

_____

_____

_____

Sweet

Fruity   Floral

Sour   Spicy

Earthy   Herbal

Woodsy

Consumed Method

Smoke	Ate	Vape	External
Rolled	Butter	Pen	Patch
Pipe	Gum		Cream
Water Pipe	Drink		Other
Blunt	Edibles		_____
Dabbed	Tincture		_____
	Oil		_____

Effects	Strength				
Peaceful	○	○	○	○	○
Sleepy	○	○	○	○	○
Pain Relief	○	○	○	○	○
Hungry	○	○	○	○	○
Uplifted	○	○	○	○	○
Creative	○	○	○	○	○

Try Again   ☐ Yes   ☐ No

Rating

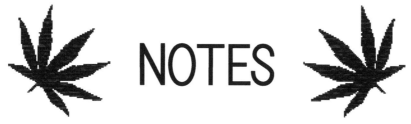

NOTES

STRAIN

Grower _____ Date _____

Acquired _____ $ _____

| THC Amount _____ CBD Oil Amount _____ | ☐ Indica | ☐ Hybrid | ☐ Sativa |

☐ Flower ☐ Edible ☐ Concentrate

Symptoms Relieved

_____
_____
_____
_____
_____

Sweet
Fruity
Floral
Sour
Spicy
Earthy
Herbal
Woodsy

Consumed Method

Smoke	Ate	Vape	External
Rolled	Butter	Pen	Patch
Pipe	Gum		Cream
Water Pipe	Drink		Other
Blunt	Edibles		_____
Dabbed	Tincture		_____
	Oil		_____

Effects — Strength

Effects	Strength				
Peaceful	○	○	○	○	○
Sleepy	○	○	○	○	○
Pain Relief	○	○	○	○	○
Hungry	○	○	○	○	○
Uplifted	○	○	○	○	○
Creative	○	○	○	○	○

Try Again ☐ Yes ☐ No

Rating 🍁 🍁 🍁 🍁 🍁

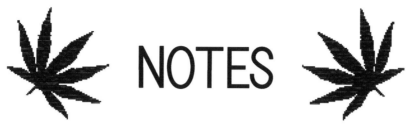

NOTES

STRAIN

Grower _____   Date _____

Acquired _____ $ _____

| THC Amount _____ | CBD Oil Amount _____ | ☐ Indica | ☐ Hybrid | ☐ Sativa |

☐ Flower   ☐ Edible   ☐ Concentrate

Symptoms Relieved

_____

_____

_____

_____

Sweet

Fruity   Floral

Sour   Spicy

Earthy   Herbal

Woodsy

Consumed Method

Smoke	Ate	Vape	External
Rolled	Butter	Pen	Patch
Pipe	Gum		Cream
Water Pipe	Drink		Other
Blunt	Edibles		_____
Dabbed	Tincture		_____
	Oil		_____

Effects	Strength				
Peaceful	○	○	○	○	○
Sleepy	○	○	○	○	○
Pain Relief	○	○	○	○	○
Hungry	○	○	○	○	○
Uplifted	○	○	○	○	○
Creative	○	○	○	○	○

Try Again   ☐ Yes   ☐ No

Rating 🌿 🌿 🌿 🌿 🌿

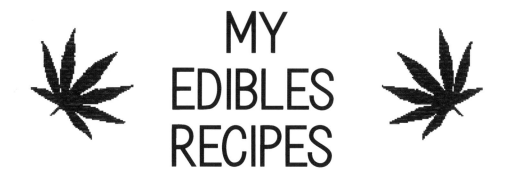

MY
EDIBLES
RECIPES

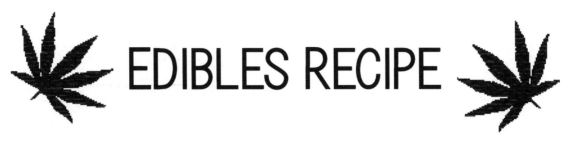

EDIBLES RECIPE

Cannabis Strain

Type   ☐ Dry   ☐ Wet

Amount Used

_____ Pinches   _____ Grams   _____ Ounces

_____ Cups   _____ Drops   _____ Teaspoons

_____ FL oz   _____ Tablespoons

Other Ingredients   Amount

Directions

Results

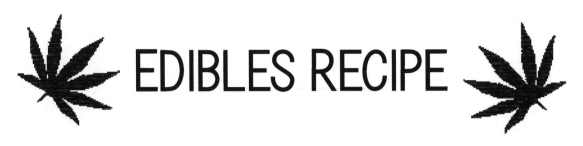

EDIBLES RECIPE

Cannabis Strain

Type   ☐ Dry   ☐ Wet

Amount Used

_____ Pinches   _____ Grams   _____ Ounces

_____ Cups   _____ Drops   _____ Teaspoons

_____ FL oz   _____ Tablespoons

Other Ingredients   Amount

Directions

Results

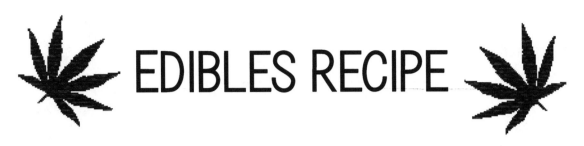

EDIBLES RECIPE

Cannabis Strain

Type ☐ Dry ☐ Wet

Amount Used

_____ Pinches _____ Grams _____ Ounces

_____ Cups _____ Drops _____ Teaspoons

_____ FL oz _____ Tablespoons

Other Ingredients   Amount

Directions

Results

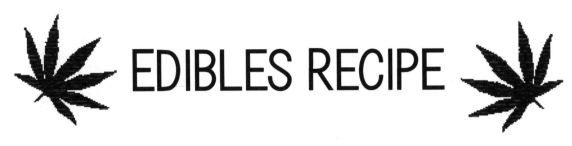

EDIBLES RECIPE

Cannabis Strain

Type   ☐ Dry   ☐ Wet

Amount Used

_____ Pinches   _____ Grams   _____ Ounces

_____ Cups   _____ Drops   _____ Teaspoons

_____ FL oz   _____ Tablespoons

Other Ingredients   Amount

Directions

Results

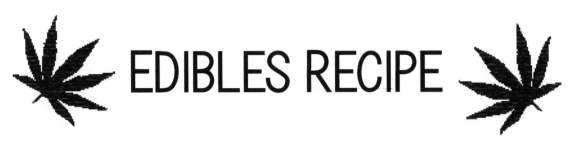

EDIBLES RECIPE

Cannabis Strain

Type ☐ Dry ☐ Wet

Amount Used

_____ Pinches _____ Grams _____ Ounces

_____ Cups _____ Drops _____ Teaspoons

_____ FL oz _____ Tablespoons

Other Ingredients   Amount

Directions

Results

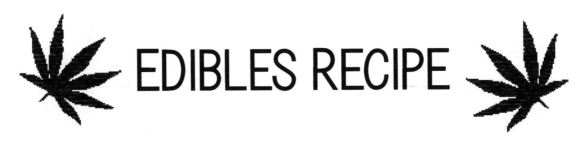

EDIBLES RECIPE

Cannabis Strain

Type ☐ Dry ☐ Wet

Amount Used

_____ Pinches   _____ Grams   _____ Ounces

_____ Cups   _____ Drops   _____ Teaspoons

_____ FL oz   _____ Tablespoons

Other Ingredients   Amount

Directions

Results

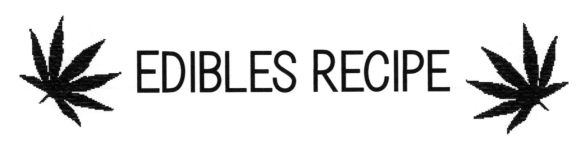

EDIBLES RECIPE

Cannabis Strain

Type   ☐ Dry   ☐ Wet

Amount Used

_____ Pinches   _____ Grams   _____ Ounces

_____ Cups   _____ Drops   _____ Teaspoons

_____ FL oz   _____ Tablespoons

Other Ingredients   Amount

Directions

Results

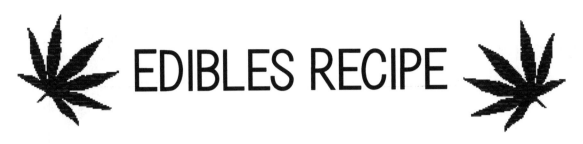

EDIBLES RECIPE

Cannabis Strain

Type   ☐ Dry   ☐ Wet

Amount Used

_____ Pinches   _____ Grams   _____ Ounces

_____ Cups   _____ Drops   _____ Teaspoons

_____ FL oz   _____ Tablespoons

Other Ingredients   Amount

Directions

Results

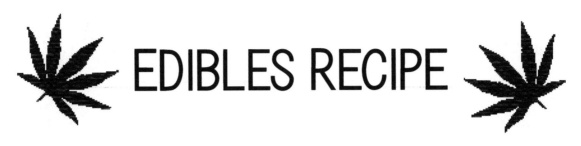

EDIBLES RECIPE

Cannabis Strain

Type   ☐ Dry   ☐ Wet

Amount Used

_____ Pinches   _____ Grams   _____ Ounces

_____ Cups   _____ Drops   _____ Teaspoons

_____ FL oz   _____ Tablespoons

Other Ingredients   Amount

Directions

Results

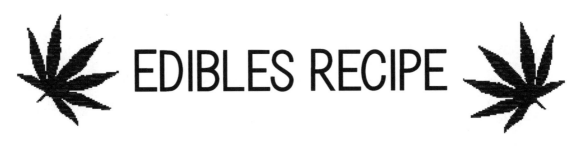

EDIBLES RECIPE

Cannabis Strain

Type   ☐ Dry   ☐ Wet

Amount Used

_____ Pinches   _____ Grams   _____ Ounces

_____ Cups   _____ Drops   _____ Teaspoons

_____ FL oz   _____ Tablespoons

Other Ingredients   Amount

Directions

Results

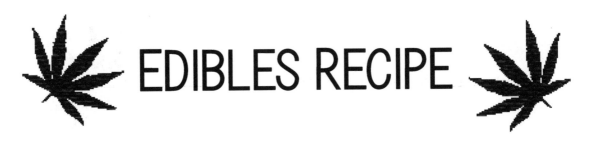

EDIBLES RECIPE

Cannabis Strain

Type ☐ Dry ☐ Wet

Amount Used

_____ Pinches _____ Grams _____ Ounces

_____ Cups _____ Drops _____ Teaspoons

_____ FL oz _____ Tablespoons

Other Ingredients   Amount

Directions

Results

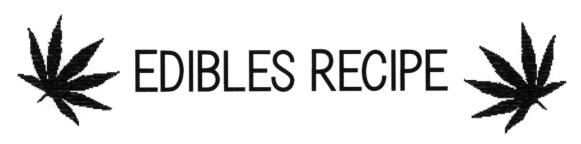

EDIBLES RECIPE

Cannabis Strain

Type ☐ Dry ☐ Wet

Amount Used

_____ Pinches   _____ Grams   _____ Ounces

_____ Cups   _____ Drops   _____ Teaspoons

_____ FL oz   _____ Tablespoons

Other Ingredients   Amount

Directions

Results

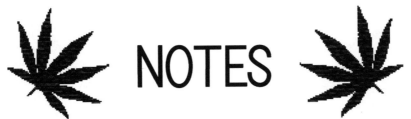

NOTES

63949707R00084